A
Monster Meeting
About Healthy Eating

Draga Stefanovic

AuthorHouse™
1663 Liberty Drive
Bloomington, IN 47403
www.authorhouse.com
Phone: 1-800-839-8640

Published by AuthorHouse 5/13/2014

ISBN: 978-1-4969-0875-9 (sc)
ISBN: 978-1-4969-0876-6 (e)

Library of Congress Control Number: 2014907894

authorHOUSE™

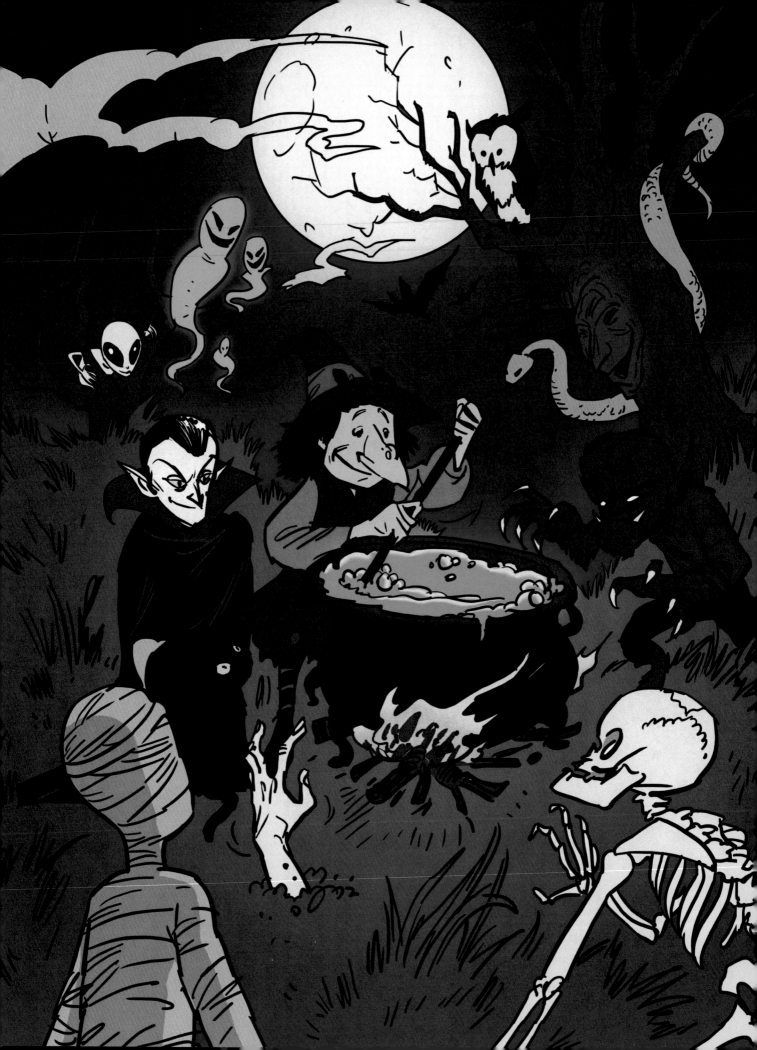

In the deep, dark woods on a cool fall night, the meeting of monsters came to order. Gathered around a huge, bubbling pot were the most fearsome, bloodthirsty, and scary monsters in history.

1

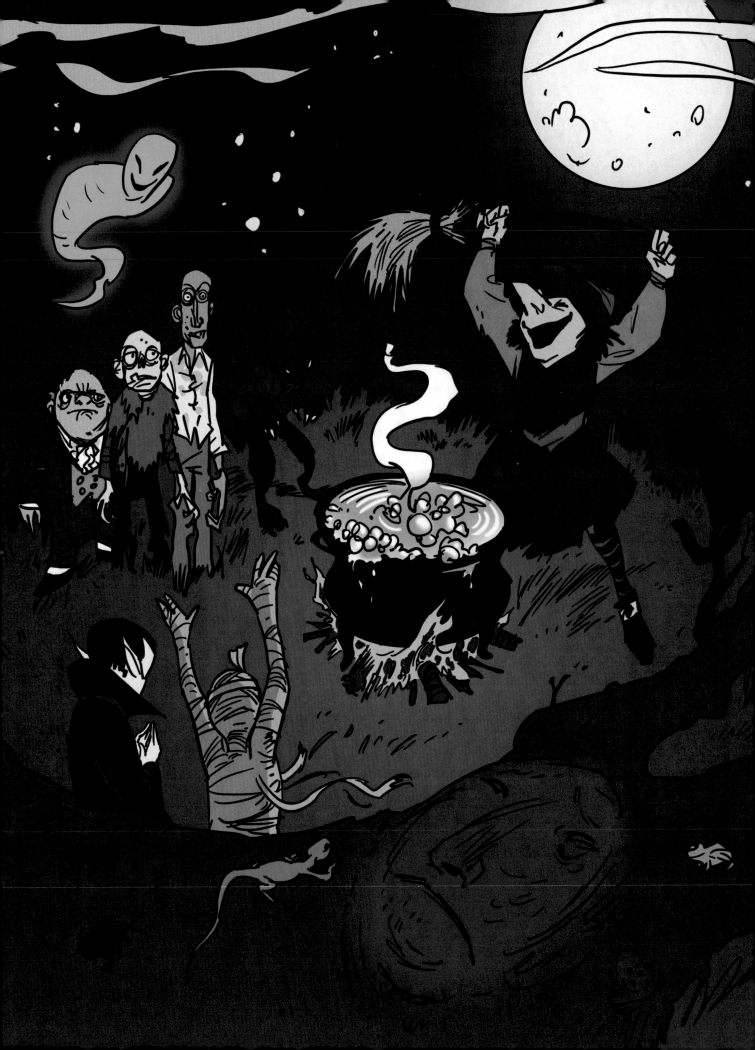

Stirring the big black pot, the wicked old witch spoke to the monster crew.

"Our goal is to conjure the most spooktactular treats ever. I hope everyone has done their monsterly best to make this Halloween one to remember!" The witch cackled and shook her broom high in the air.

All the monsters yelped and danced with delight.

2

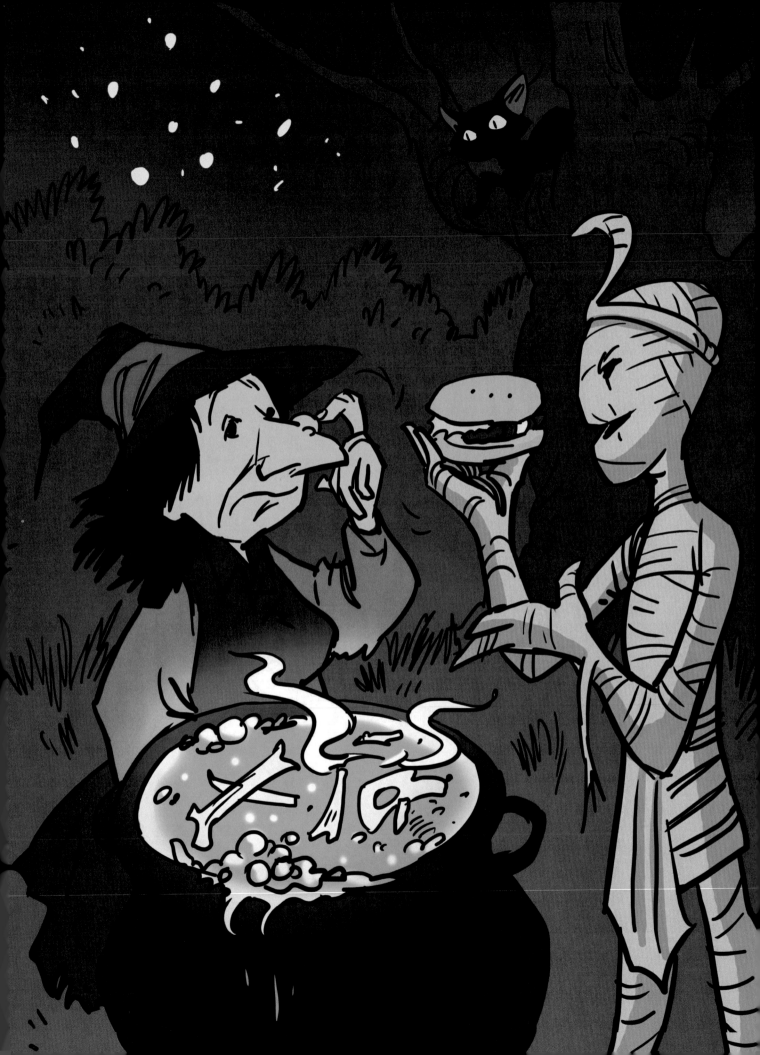

"All right, everyone," said the witch. "Let's get started. Mummy, what did you wrap up?"

"I brought bacon cheeseburgers and chocolate malts. Yum! They taste so good!"

The monsters cheered and clapped in favor.

"Hmm, cheeseburgers. High in fat, aren't they?" asked the witch. "I'm not so sure. It doesn't seem right." The witch scratched at her wart and wrinkled her nose. "I suppose they'll do. Throw them in."

The mummy did, and the brewing pot was stirred.

3

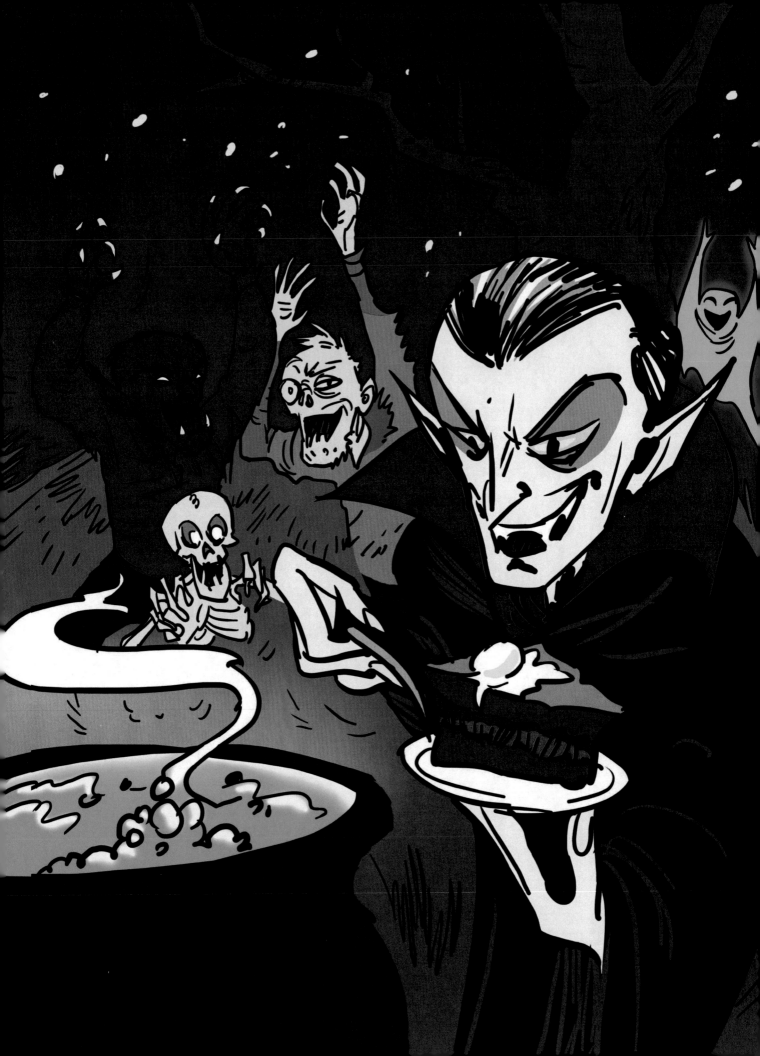

"Vampire, what about you? What did you scare up?"

"Red-velvet cake and cherry suckers. They
are wonderfully sweet and moist!"

The monsters howled and stomped in excitement.

"Carbs? You brought sugary snacks and cake to this meeting?
You've got to be kidding!" the witch scolded. "I just don't know.
It doesn't seem right." The witch rubbed her head and made
a mean face. "I suppose they'll do. Throw them in."

The vampire did, and the brewing pot was stirred.

4

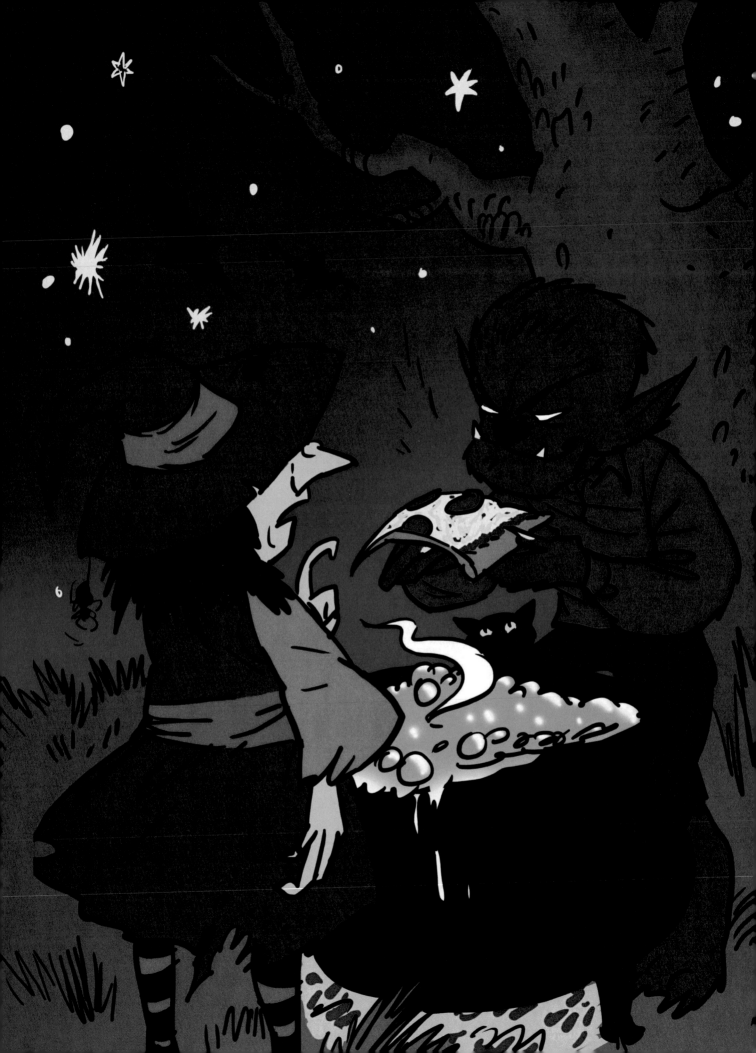

"Werewolf, my good friend, what did you dig up?"

"Stuffed-crust pizza and a family order of breadsticks;
both are filling and one of my favorite meals!"

The monsters yipped and yapped in approval.

"Dripping cheese, carbs, and fat." The witch smirked and rolled
her eyes. "I just don't know. It doesn't seem right." The witch
curled her nose and made a sour face. "I suppose they'll do.

Throw them in."

The werewolf did, and the brewing pot was stirred.

5

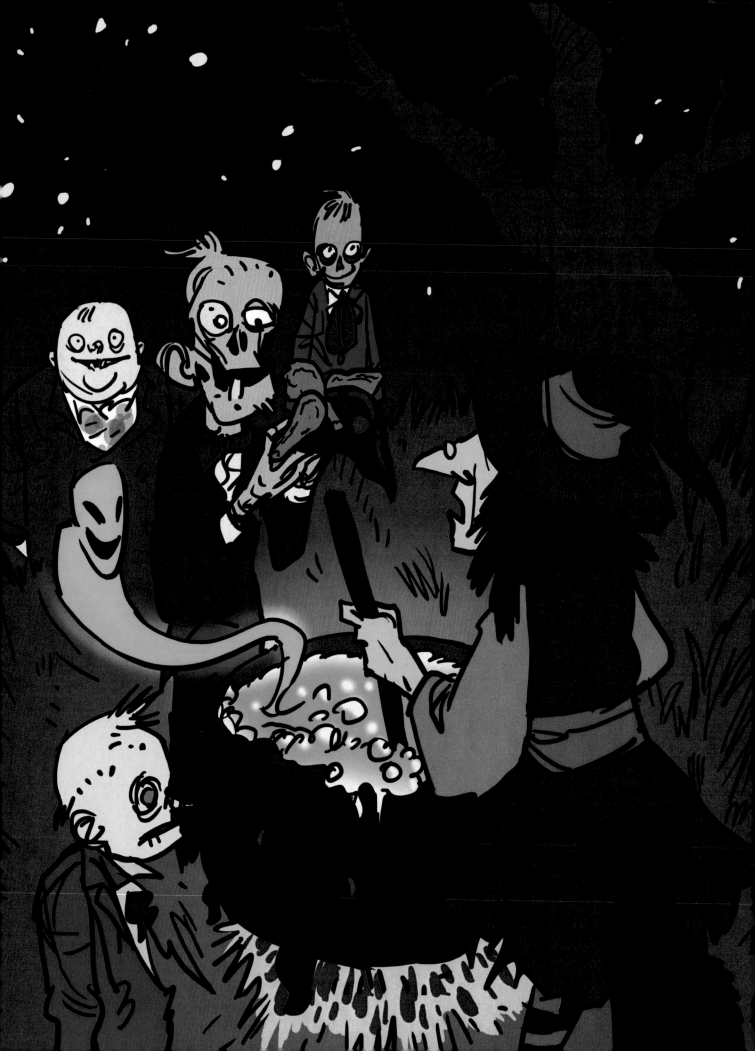

"Zombie, what did you drag in?"

"Fresh liver and fried chicken. Oh, I love them so!"

The monsters shouted and jumped in support.

"Again with the fat," the witch said. "And isn't organ meat high in cholesterol? Ugh! We seem to be in a rut here. I just don't know. It doesn't seem right." The witch moaned and shook her head. "I suppose they'll do. Throw them in."

The zombie did, and the brewing pot was stirred.

6

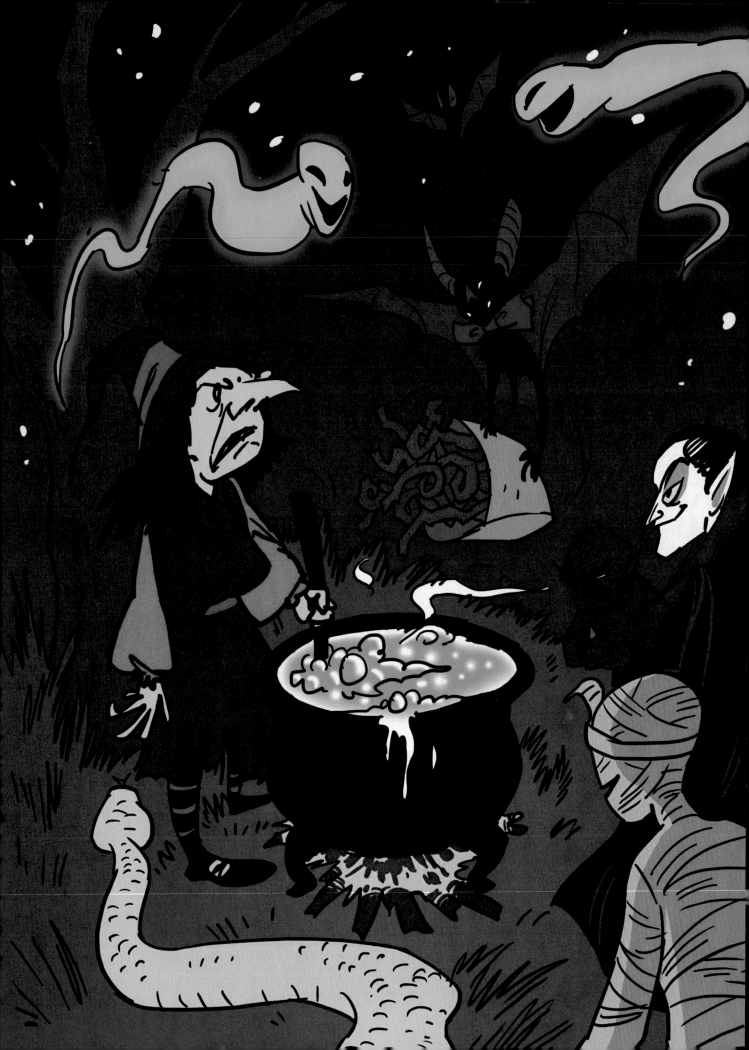

"Mr. Bat, please tell me you have something
better to offer," pleaded the witch.

"Well," said the bat with a shiver, "I picked up curly fries
and cheese curds. They're light and easy to carry!"

The monsters huddled together and didn't say a word.

The witch paused, staring blankly at the monster crew
before her, and threw her hands in the air. "Why not?"
sneered the witch with sarcasm. "Throw them in."

Mr. Bat did, and the brewing pot was stirred.

7

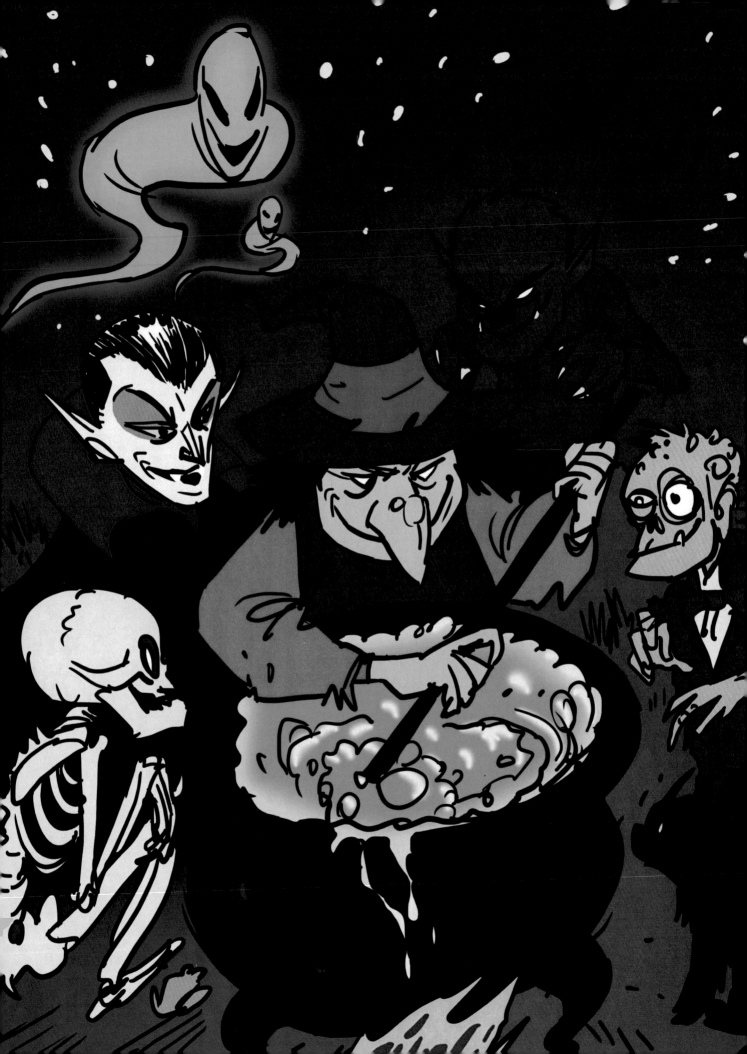

All the monsters glared at the witch, unhappy
with her condescending tone.

"And what did you bring that's so great?" the monsters demanded.

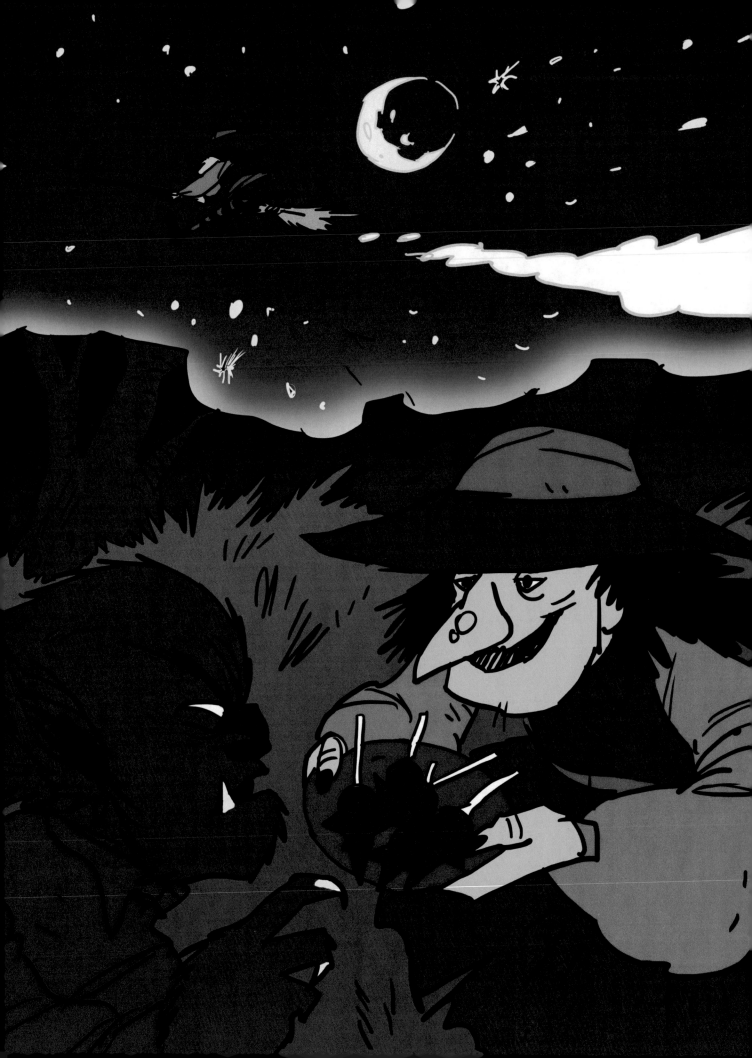

"Who, me?" said the witch.

"Yes, you!" the monsters ordered.

"Well, I've been very busy with work these days," explained the witch. "So the other night, I flew to the store, totally unnoticed, and picked up the cutest witches on a stick and bite-sized candy bars!"

9

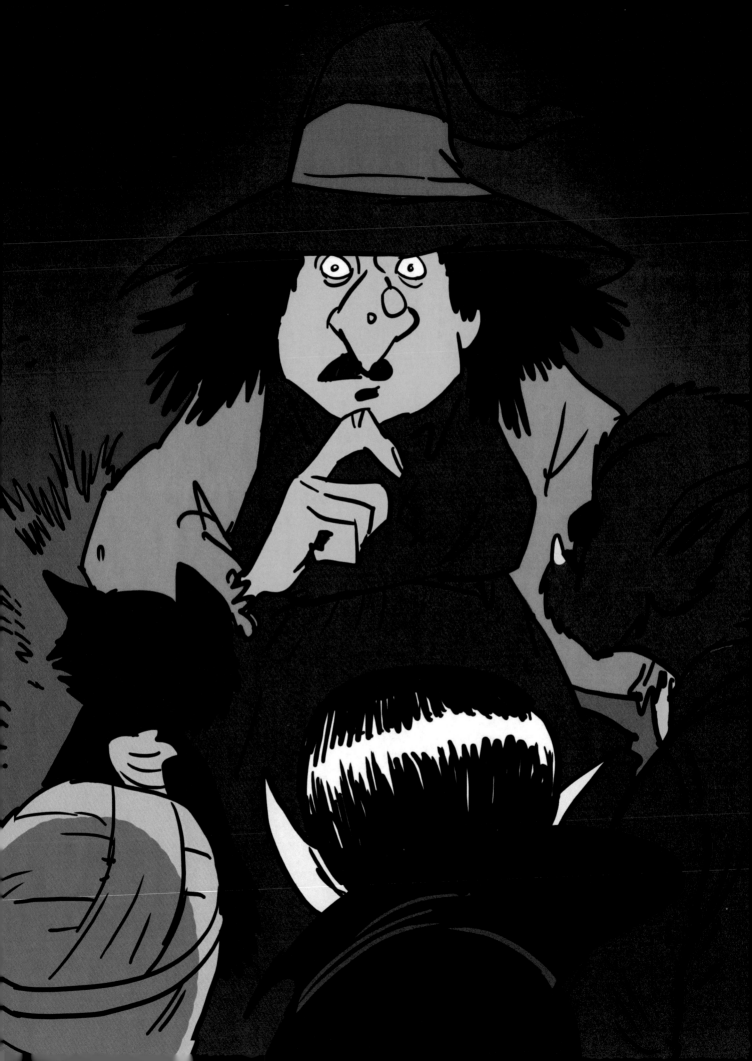

The witch peeked out from under her hat,
waiting for the monsters' approval.

"Candy bars and witches on a stick?" said the monsters, "Is that a joke?"

10

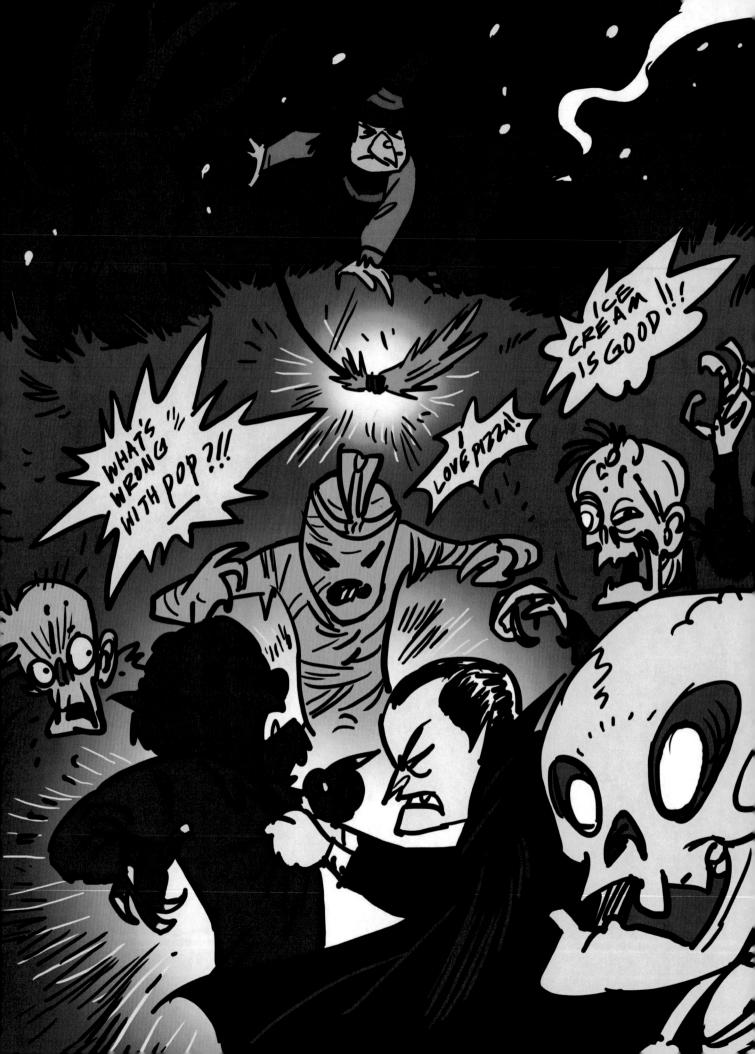

Then all the monsters began to quarrel over
whose Halloween treats were the best.

The witch slammed her broom handle to the ground, straightened her hat,
and shouted, "Let's all just calm down! Good grief, we're acting like a bunch
of goblins! We've all been brainwashed by fast food and junky snacks!"

11

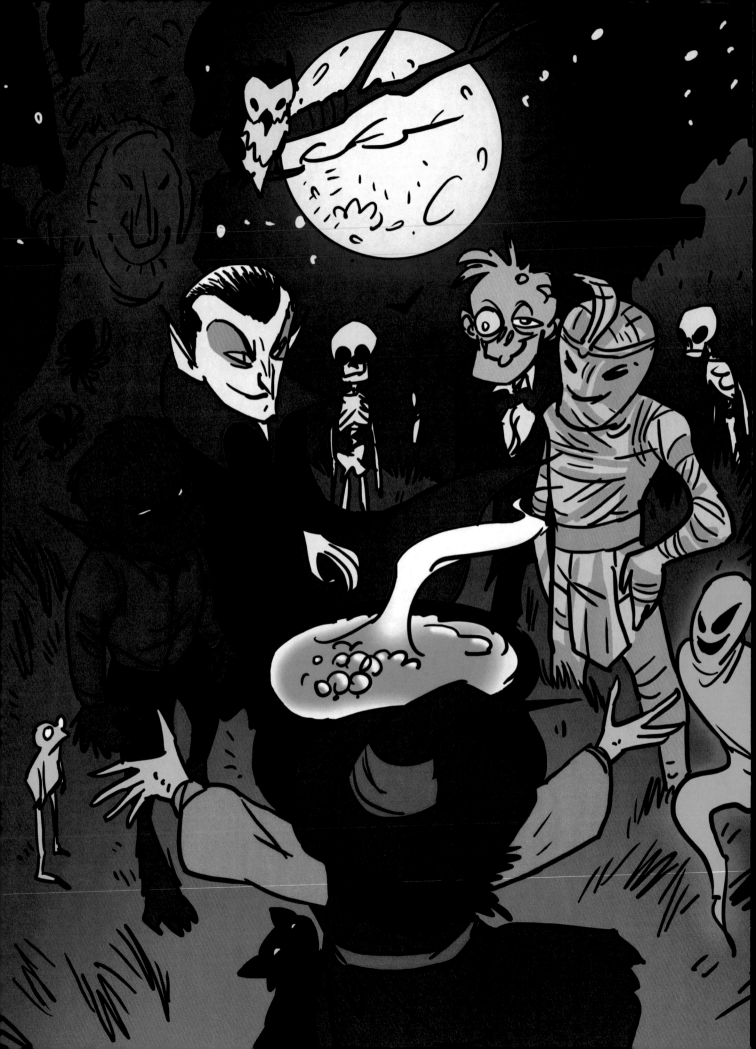

Suddenly, the monsters all looked sad and seemed to understand how poor their eating habits had become.

So with good health on their minds, the monster crew worked together to make a witch's brew worth howling over: leg of frog, pumpkin and spice, rotted root, spider, and web.

"Yum! This will be so good!" they all chanted.

And a healthy Halloween tradition began.

1. What kind of food did the monsters bring to the meeting?

2. Why did the witch get so upset?

3. How did the monsters develop poor eating habits?

4. What are some healthy snacks the monsters
   could have brought to the meeting?

5. What are some things we can eat to help keep our bodies strong?

6. What can we do to stay healthy?

13

About the Book:

A Monster Meeting about Healthy Eating is an educational book about a group of monsters that have developed an unhealthy appetite for fast food and junky snacks. Led by a witch, the monsters meet and try to conjure the best Halloween treats ever. As the story unfolds, the monsters realize how their eating habits have changed and work together to promote good health. The book is designed for teachers and parents to help children think about and discuss healthy choices for meals and snacks.

Printed in the United States
By Bookmasters